SCIATICA RELIEF

Effective Exercises to Alleviate
Pain, Improve Mobility, and
Regain Your Life

Dr. Raymond F. Bernard

TABLE OF CONTENTS

CHAPTER 1

Introduction to Sciatica

When it comes to understanding the challenges of sciatica, it's essential to begin with the basics. So, let's dive into Chapter 1, where we'll take a closer look at what sciatica is, why it occurs, and why exercise plays a pivotal role in managing this condition.

The Mystery of Sciatica:

Imagine the human body as a complex network of roads and

highways. Among these intricate pathways is a major nerve called the sciatic nerve. This nerve starts in the lower back and travels down through the buttocks and legs. Its job is to transmit signals between the brain and the lower body, making everything from walking to feeling sensations possible.

Now, what happens when this nerve encounters trouble? This is where sciatica makes its appearance. Sciatica isn't a condition on its own; rather, it's a symptom of an underlying issue. It occurs when there's pressure or irritation on the sciatic nerve, leading to pain, discomfort, and often a tingling sensation that radiates down the leg.

Peeling Back the Layers:

To truly grasp sciatica's impact, let's delve a bit deeper. Imagine you're leaning against a wall, and a misaligned brick is poking into your back. Over time, that tiny brick can cause discomfort, and the pain might even spread to your arm. Similarly, in the world of sciatica, various factors like a herniated disc, bone spurs, or even muscle tightness can apply pressure to the sciatic nerve, resulting in pain that follows the nerve's path.

Sciatica pain isn't uniform; it can vary from a mild ache to an intense burning sensation or sharp jolts. It's as unique as a fingerprint, varying from person to person. However, it often shares one common aspect: its potential to disrupt your daily life. Simple tasks like sitting, standing, or walking can become challenging endeavors. This is where our journey into sciatica exercise begins.

The Exercise Connection:

As we move on in this chapter, it's important to address the role of exercise in managing sciatica. You might wonder, "Why exercise? Can't I just rest and wait for the pain to subside?" While rest has its place, exercise offers a remarkable array of benefits that can't be overlooked.

Exercise is a powerful tool for managing sciatica for several reasons. First, it helps to increase blood flow and oxygen delivery to the affected area, promoting healing and reducing inflammation. Second, specific exercises can target the muscles and structures around the sciatic nerve, helping to alleviate the pressure and tension that contribute to the pain. Third, regular exercise can enhance flexibility and strength, creating a supportive environment for the spine and nerves.

However, it's important to understand that not all exercises are created equal. Just as you wouldn't use a sledgehammer to fix a delicate watch, you need the right exercises to address sciatica effectively. This is where this book comes into play – to guide you through a tailored exercise regimen designed to target sciatica at its root.

Setting the Stage:

Before we jump into the exercises themselves, it's vital to get the lay of the land. By understanding your body and the specific challenges you face, you can approach your exercise routine with confidence and clarity. This means assessing your current fitness level, understanding any limitations or medical conditions, and knowing when it's appropriate to seek professional advice.

In addition, setting realistic goals is crucial. While we'd all love a quick fix, sciatica management is a journey, not a sprint. By setting achievable goals, you'll be more motivated to stick with your exercise routine and experience the gradual improvements that come with consistent effort.

As we conclude this chapter, remember that sciatica isn't a life sentence. While it might seem overwhelming now, the journey to managing and alleviating your pain is within reach. With the right knowledge, exercises, and dedication, you're taking the first steps toward regaining control of your life and saying goodbye to the grip of sciatica. The chapters ahead will guide you through the ins and outs of sciatica exercises, equipping you with the tools to overcome this challenge and embrace a life of comfort and mobility.

CHAPTER 2

Understanding Sciatica Pain

Welcome to Chapter 2, where we're about to uncover the intricate world of sciatica pain. Let's delve into the depths of what this pain is, how it works, and why it's so crucial to comprehend its nuances as we navigate the path toward relief.

Unveiling the Sciatic Nerve:

Imagine your sciatic nerve as the body's grand communication highway. Just like a major freeway connects different cities, this nerve links the lower body to the brain. Starting from the lower back, it journeys through the buttocks, down the back of the legs, and finally reaches the feet. It's responsible for sensation, movement, and function in this entire region.

Now, imagine construction blocking a highway. Traffic jams, delays, and frustration follow suit. Similarly, when something disrupts the sciatic nerve's smooth operation, we encounter sciatica pain. But what could cause such a disruption?

The Origins of Sciatica Pain:

The most common trigger for sciatica is the pressure or irritation applied to the nerve. This pressure often arises from herniated discs, which are like cushions between the vertebrae that can bulge or rupture. When they do, they might press against the sciatic nerve, triggering the infamous pain that shoots down the leg.

Another potential culprit is spinal stenosis – a narrowing of the spinal canal. This narrowing can squeeze the sciatic nerve, causing discomfort. Bone spurs, which are overgrowths of bone, can also encroach on the nerve's territory, leading to pain.

Yet another factor is muscle tightness. Muscles, when overly tense, can compress the sciatic nerve, causing pain to radiate through the leg. These triggers, among others, create a symphony of sensations that characterize sciatica pain.

The Spectrum of Pain:

Just as no two fingerprints are the same, sciatica pain varies from person to person. It can range from a dull ache to a burning sensation, a throbbing discomfort, or even intense electric-like jolts. For some, the pain is intermittent, flaring up on occasion. For others, it's a constant companion, shadowing their every move.

The nature of the pain largely depends on factors like the underlying cause, the degree of pressure on the nerve, and an individual's pain threshold. Regardless of the specifics, one thing remains universal: sciatica pain often follows the nerve's path, traveling from the lower back down through the buttocks and the back of the leg, sometimes extending all the way to the foot.

Impact on Daily Life:

Perhaps the most poignant aspect of sciatica pain is its ability to disrupt even the simplest of tasks. Picture trying to enjoy a leisurely walk with a pebble in your shoe – the discomfort can consume your attention and overshadow the beauty of the moment. Sciatica pain operates similarly, casting a shadow over activities as basic as sitting, standing, or walking.

Sitting can be especially challenging, as pressure on the nerve is often intensified in this position. Standing might bring relief to some, but for others, it's a reminder of the constant discomfort. Even lying down doesn't guarantee escape from the pain, as finding a comfortable sleeping position can become an ongoing battle.

Navigating the Journey:

Understanding the complexities of sciatica pain is the first step toward effective management. It's important to recognize that while the pain can be overwhelming, it doesn't define who you are. It's a challenge, but one that can be overcome.

In the upcoming chapters, we'll explore how exercise, specifically tailored to your needs, can alleviate the pressure on the sciatic nerve, soothe muscle tension, and restore mobility. Armed with a deeper understanding of the pain's origins, you'll be better equipped to appreciate the exercises that follow and their potential to lead you toward a life with less pain and more freedom.

So, remember that while sciatica pain might have its grip on you right now, knowledge and action are your allies. As we move forward, keep in mind that the pain is not your identity – it's a signal from your body that something needs attention. With this newfound knowledge, you're ready to venture into the world of sciatica exercise, armed with a deeper appreciation of the journey ahead.

CHAPTER 3

The Science of Exercise and Sciatica

Welcome to Chapter 3, where we delve into the science behind exercise and its pivotal role in managing sciatica. Understanding why exercise is a cornerstone of sciatica relief is essential for appreciating its potential and committing to a structured exercise regimen. Let's embark on this journey of knowledge and empowerment.

The Healing Power of Exercise:

Imagine your body as a finely tuned machine, each part serving a specific purpose. Just like a car needs regular maintenance to function at its best, your body requires movement and activity to thrive. This is where exercise comes into play. It's not just about aesthetics or fitness; it's about maintaining the health and functionality of your muscles, joints, and nerves.

Now, let's focus on the sciatic nerve. When pressure or irritation affects it, it can trigger the pain and discomfort known as sciatica. Exercise is a potent tool in addressing this condition because it serves several critical functions in the healing process:

1. **Increased Blood Flow:** Exercise boosts circulation, promoting the delivery of oxygen and nutrients to the affected area. This helps in reducing inflammation and facilitating the healing of damaged tissues.

2. **Muscle and Joint Mobility:** Specific exercises can target the muscles surrounding the sciatic

nerve, alleviating tension and pressure. They also enhance the flexibility of the spine and joints, which can prevent further irritation of the nerve.

3. **Strength and Support:** Strengthening exercises help build a supportive structure for the spine. A strong core and back muscles provide stability, reducing the risk of future sciatica episodes.

4. **Endorphin Release:** Exercise triggers the release of endorphins, the body's natural pain relievers. This can offer immediate relief

from sciatica discomfort and contribute to an improved mood.

Types of Exercises for Sciatica Relief:

Not all exercises are created equal, especially when it comes to sciatica relief. The key is to engage in exercises that specifically target the underlying causes of your pain. Here are some types of exercises commonly recommended for sciatica:

1. **Stretching and Flexibility Exercises:** These exercises focus on

elongating and loosening the muscles and structures that may be compressing the sciatic nerve. They often involve gentle movements that aim to relieve tension.

2. **Strengthening Exercises:** These exercises primarily focus on building the strength of the muscles that support the spine and pelvis. A strong core, for example, can significantly reduce the strain on the sciatic nerve.

3. **Cardiovascular Exercises:** Engaging in cardiovascular activities, like

walking, swimming, or cycling, can improve overall health and circulation. These exercises help in reducing inflammation and promoting healing.

4. **Low-Impact Exercises:** Especially beneficial for individuals with severe pain, low-impact exercises like water aerobics or elliptical training provide a workout without putting excess stress on the joints.

5. **Yoga and Pilates:** These mind-body practices emphasize flexibility, balance, and core strength,

making them excellent choices for sciatica management. Many yoga poses and Pilates exercises specifically target the lower back and hip region.

6. **Physical Therapy:** Often recommended for severe or chronic cases, physical therapy provides a tailored approach to sciatica relief. A physical therapist can assess your condition and design a customized exercise plan.

The Timing and Consistency Factor:

The benefits of exercise for sciatica relief are most pronounced when it becomes a consistent part of your routine. Regular exercise helps in maintaining the improvements you achieve and prevents future episodes of sciatica. It's like brushing your teeth – daily maintenance is key to preventing cavities.

However, it's equally important to recognize that exercise should be approached with caution. If you're currently experiencing severe pain or have certain medical conditions, it's essential to consult with a healthcare professional before starting any exercise regimen. They can provide guidance on exercises that are safe and appropriate for your specific situation.

Why Exercise is a Long-Term Solution:

One of the remarkable aspects of exercise in sciatica management is its potential to provide long-term relief. While medications may offer temporary comfort, exercise addresses the root causes of sciatica, promoting healing and preventing future flare-ups. It's an investment in your future well-being.

By regularly engaging in exercises tailored to your condition, you can build strength, flexibility, and resilience in your body. Over time, you'll likely notice a reduction in the frequency and intensity of sciatica episodes. Plus, the overall health benefits of exercise, such as improved cardiovascular health and enhanced mood, are valuable additions to your life.

Closing Thoughts:

As we wrap up Chapter 3, remember that exercise isn't just a recommendation; it's a powerful tool for regaining control over your life in the face of sciatica. By understanding the science behind exercise's role in managing sciatica, you're better equipped to appreciate its significance.

In the chapters that follow, we'll delve deeper into specific exercises tailored to address the unique challenges of sciatica. With the right knowledge and commitment, you'll embark on a journey toward greater comfort, mobility, and freedom from the grip of sciatica pain. Your body has incredible potential for healing and resilience, and exercise is your trusted companion on this path to recovery.

CHAPTER 4

Preparing for Exercise

Welcome to Chapter 4, where we're about to lay the groundwork for your sciatica exercise journey. Just as a well-built foundation supports a sturdy house, preparing your body and mind for exercise is essential for maximizing the benefits and minimizing risks. Let's dive into the crucial steps to take before diving into your exercise routine.

The Importance of Assessment:

Before you embark on any exercise program, it's essential to take a step back and assess where you currently stand. Think of this as a GPS guiding you to your destination. By understanding your starting point, you can chart a more effective course.

Assessing your current fitness level involves understanding your strengths, limitations, and any existing medical conditions. Are there certain movements that trigger your sciatica pain? Are there activities you've been avoiding due to discomfort? By identifying these factors, you can tailor your exercise routine to avoid exacerbating your pain while targeting the areas that need attention.

Seeking Professional Guidance:

While empowerment is a crucial part of this journey, there are times when professional guidance is invaluable. If your sciatica pain is severe or if you have existing medical conditions, it's wise to consult a healthcare professional before beginning any exercise regimen. This could be your primary care physician, a physical therapist, or a specialist.

These professionals can provide a thorough evaluation of your condition and suggest exercises that are safe and appropriate for your specific situation. They'll also guide you on how to modify exercises if necessary and provide strategies to prevent overexertion.

Setting Realistic Goals:

Imagine you're planning a road trip. It's essential to know your destination and how long it'll take to get there. Similarly, when it comes to exercise, setting realistic goals is key. Acknowledge that sciatica relief is a journey, not an overnight sensation. Establishing attainable goals ensures that you're motivated and committed for the long haul.

Your goals could range from reducing the frequency of sciatica episodes to improving your flexibility or being able to perform specific activities without pain. These objectives will serve as a roadmap, guiding your exercise routine and tracking your progress.

Understanding Pain Signals:

Pain is like your body's alarm system, alerting you when something needs attention. However, in the context of exercise for sciatica, understanding the difference between productive discomfort and harmful pain is crucial.

Productive discomfort might feel like stretching a tight muscle – it's uncomfortable but not sharp or jolting. Harmful pain, on the other hand, is sharp, shooting, or intense. If you experience harmful pain during an exercise, stop immediately. It's your body's way of saying "this isn't right." This is another reason why professional guidance is so important – they can help you distinguish between discomfort that leads to improvement and pain that should be avoided.

The Importance of Consistency:

Imagine planting a garden. The more consistently you water and care for the plants, the better they'll grow. Similarly, the benefits of exercise for sciatica relief are most pronounced when it becomes a consistent part of your routine.

Consistency doesn't mean pushing through pain; it means dedicating time regularly to exercises that are appropriate for your condition. This gradual, sustained effort helps build strength, flexibility, and resilience over time. It's like a savings account for your health – small deposits accumulate into significant benefits.

Listening to Your Body:

Your body is your most reliable guide on this journey. Just as a navigator listens to the GPS, you should listen to your body's signals. If a certain exercise feels uncomfortable or worsens your pain, it's okay to modify or skip it. Flexibility in your routine is essential – what works for one person might not work for another.

Remember that this journey is about progress, not perfection. Some days might be more challenging than others, and that's okay. Celebrate the small victories and be kind to yourself on the days when progress is slower.

Final Thoughts:

Chapter 4 has equipped you with the tools needed to lay a strong foundation for your sciatica exercise journey. By assessing your fitness level, seeking professional guidance, setting realistic goals, understanding pain signals, and prioritizing consistency, you're ready to embark on the next phase.

In the upcoming chapters, we'll dive into specific stretches, exercises, and routines that cater to your needs. With your foundation in place, you're well-prepared to make the most of the exercises that follow. Your commitment, combined with knowledge and careful planning, will lead you to a life with less pain and greater mobility. So, let's move forward with confidence and determination, knowing that you're taking steps toward regaining control over your well-being.

CHAPTER 5

Stretching and Flexibility Exercises

Welcome to Chapter 5, where we'll delve into the world of stretching and flexibility exercises tailored to alleviate sciatica pain. Stretching is like opening the curtains to let in the morning sun; it helps ease stiffness, reduce muscle tension, and pave the way for increased mobility. In this chapter, we'll explore the importance of stretching, its benefits for sciatica, and some specific exercises to get you started.

The Importance of Stretching:

Imagine your muscles as elastic bands. When these bands are well-stretched and flexible, they can move smoothly without causing strain or pulling on surrounding structures like the sciatic nerve. However, when these bands become tight and inflexible, they can tug and put pressure on the sciatic nerve, triggering or exacerbating pain.

Stretching is the key to maintaining the suppleness of your muscles and joints. It helps improve your range of motion, reduce stiffness, and ease muscle tension. For individuals with sciatica, it's a vital component of pain management because it directly addresses the factors that contribute to sciatic nerve irritation.

Benefits of Stretching for Sciatica:

Stretching exercises offer a host of benefits for individuals dealing with sciatica:

1. **Tension Relief:** Stretching helps release tension in the muscles around the sciatic nerve, reducing the pressure on the nerve and alleviating pain.

2. **Improved Flexibility:** Regular stretching gradually increases your muscle and joint flexibility, making it easier to move without discomfort.

3. **Increased Blood Flow:** Stretching enhances blood circulation, delivering essential nutrients and oxygen to the affected area, which can aid in healing.

4. **Reduced Risk of Injury:** Flexible muscles are less prone to injury, which is crucial for individuals with sciatica, as injury can exacerbate their condition.

5. **Enhanced Posture:** Stretching exercises that target the lower back and core can improve posture, reducing strain on the spine and sciatic nerve.

Pre-Stretching Guidelines:

Before we dive into specific stretching exercises, let's establish some essential guidelines to ensure a safe and effective stretching routine:

1. **Warm-Up:** It's crucial to warm up your muscles before stretching. Gentle activities like walking or light cycling for 5-10 minutes increase blood flow and prepare your muscles for stretching.

2. **Maintain Consistency:** Stretching is most effective when performed regularly. Aim to stretch daily or at least several times a week to experience significant benefits.

3. **Hold, Don't Bounce:** When stretching, avoid bouncing or jerking movements. Instead, hold each stretch for 15-30 seconds, allowing your muscles to relax gradually.

4. **Focus on Breathing:** Pay attention to your breathing while stretching. Inhale deeply as you prepare for the stretch, and exhale slowly as you ease into it. Deep, controlled breathing can help relax your muscles.

5. **No Pain:** Stretching should never cause pain. You should feel a gentle pulling

sensation, but if you experience pain, stop immediately. Pain is your body's way of saying the stretch is too intense.

Stretching Exercises for Sciatica:

Now, let's explore some stretching exercises specifically designed to target areas that commonly contribute to sciatica pain. As you perform these stretches, remember to start slowly, hold each stretch for the recommended time, and never force your body into a position that causes pain.

1. **Knee-to-Chest Stretch:**

   - Lie on your back with both knees bent.
   - Slowly bring one knee toward your chest, holding it with both hands.
   - Hold for 15-30 seconds, then switch to the other knee.
   - Repeat this stretch 2-3 times for each leg.

2. **Piriformis Stretch:**

   - Begin by sitting with one leg extended straight.
   - Cross your other leg over the extended leg,

placing your foot flat on the floor.

- o Gently pull your bent knee toward your chest until you feel a stretch in the buttocks.
- o Hold for 15-30 seconds and switch sides.
- o Repeat 2-3 times for each side.

3. **Hamstring Stretch:**

- o Sit on the floor with one leg extended and the other bent so that the sole of your foot touches the inner thigh of the extended leg.

o Reach for your toes on the extended leg, keeping your back straight.

o Hold for 15-30 seconds, then switch to the other leg.

o Repeat 2-3 times for each leg.

4. **Cat-Cow Stretch:**

o Start on your hands and knees in a tabletop position.

o Inhale as you arch your back, lifting your head and tailbone (Cow Pose).

- Exhale as you round your back, tucking your chin and tailbone (Cat Pose).
- Repeat this sequence for 30 seconds to 1 minute.

5. **Child's Pose:**

- Kneel on the floor with your big toes touching and knees apart.
- Sit back on your heels and extend your arms forward on the floor.
- Rest your forehead on the ground and hold for 30 seconds to 1 minute.

Chapter 5 has introduced you to the world of stretching and flexibility exercises tailored to alleviate sciatica pain. Stretching is a powerful tool for managing sciatica by reducing muscle tension, increasing flexibility, and promoting blood flow to the affected area. As you incorporate these exercises into your routine, remember the importance of consistency, proper warm-up, and listening to your body's signals.

In the chapters ahead, we'll explore strengthening exercises, cardiovascular activities, and low-impact options to create a well-rounded approach to sciatica management. By combining these exercises with a dedication to stretching and flexibility, you'll be on your way to regaining control over your life and experiencing less pain and greater mobility. So, let's continue this journey with optimism and determination, knowing that each stretch brings you one step closer to a more comfortable and active lifestyle.

CHAPTER 6

Strengthening Exercises

Welcome to Chapter 6, where we'll dive into the world of strengthening exercises designed to build a strong and supportive foundation for managing sciatica. Think of strengthening as constructing a sturdy bridge – it helps provide stability, reduce strain on the sciatic nerve, and protect against future pain episodes. In this chapter, we'll explore the significance of strength training, its benefits for sciatica, and specific exercises to help you build resilience.

The Importance of Strength Training:

Imagine your body as a building, with your muscles as the framework. A well-structured frame ensures stability and support for the entire structure. Similarly, strengthening exercises provide the necessary framework for your body to function optimally.

When you have sciatica, it's crucial to address the muscle imbalances and weaknesses that can contribute to your pain. Strengthening exercises target the muscles of the lower back, core, hips, and legs, which are essential for maintaining proper posture, reducing strain on the spine, and supporting the sciatic nerve.

Benefits of Strengthening for Sciatica:

Engaging in a regular strength training routine offers numerous advantages for individuals dealing with sciatica:

1. **Muscle Support:** Strong muscles in the lower back and core provide essential

support to the spine, reducing pressure on the sciatic nerve.

2. **Improved Posture:** Strengthening exercises help you maintain good posture, preventing excessive stress on the lower back and reducing the risk of pain.

3. **Stability:** A strong core stabilizes the spine and pelvis, reducing the risk of misalignment that can trigger sciatica.

4. **Pain Prevention:** Strengthening exercises can help prevent future episodes of sciatica by addressing

underlying weaknesses and imbalances.

5. **Enhanced Functionality:** As your strength increases, you'll find it easier to perform daily activities without pain or discomfort.

Pre-Strengthening Guidelines:

Before we delve into the specific strengthening exercises, let's establish some important guidelines to ensure a safe and effective strength training routine:

1. **Proper Form:** Maintaining proper form is crucial to

prevent injury and ensure that you're targeting the intended muscle groups. If you're unsure about your form, consider consulting a fitness professional.

2. **Start with Low Resistance:** When beginning a strength training program, it's essential to start with low resistance (lightweights or resistance bands) and gradually increase as your strength improves.

3. **Balanced Approach:** Ensure that you work on both sides of your body

evenly. Imbalances can lead to further problems, so strive for symmetry in your strengthening routine.

4. **Rest and Recovery:** Adequate rest between strength training sessions is essential for muscle recovery and growth. Aim for at least 48 hours of rest between sessions targeting the same muscle group.

5. **Warm-Up:** Just as with stretching, it's crucial to warm up before strength training to prepare your muscles. Incorporate

dynamic stretches and light cardio for 5-10 minutes.

Strengthening Exercises for Sciatica:

Now, let's explore some strengthening exercises that specifically target the muscles involved in sciatica management. As you perform these exercises, remember to start with low resistance and focus on proper form.

1. **Bridges:**
   - Lie on your back with your knees bent and feet flat on the floor.

- Tighten your abdominal muscles and lift your hips off the ground until your body forms a straight line from your shoulders to your knees.
- Hold for a few seconds, then lower your hips back down.
- Repeat 10-15 times for 2-3 sets.

2. **Planks:**

- Start in a push-up position with your elbows directly under your shoulders and your body in a straight line from head to heels.

- o Engage your core muscles and hold this position for as long as you can, aiming for 20-30 seconds initially and gradually increasing over time.
- o Perform 2-3 sets.

3. **Bird-Dog Exercise:**

- o Begin on your hands and knees in a tabletop position.
- o Extend your right arm forward and your left leg backward, keeping

them parallel to the floor.

- o Hold for a few seconds, then return to the starting position.
- o Switch to the opposite arm and leg.
- o Repeat 10-15 times for 2-3 sets on each side.

4. **Wall Sits:**

- o Stand with your back against a wall and your feet hip-width apart.
- o Slide down the wall, bending your knees until they are at a 90-degree angle.

- o Hold this position for as long as you can, aiming for 20-30 seconds initially and gradually increasing over time.
- o Perform 2-3 sets.

5. **Pelvic Tilts:**

- o Lie on your back with your knees bent and feet flat on the floor.
- o Tighten your abdominal muscles and gently tilt your pelvis upward, flattening your lower back against the floor.

- o Hold for a few seconds, then release.
- o Repeat 10-15 times for 2-3 sets.

Closing Thoughts:

Chapter 6 has delved into the world of strengthening exercises tailored to build a strong foundation for managing sciatica. Remember that strength training is not about lifting heavyweights but about creating balance and support in your body.

As you incorporate these exercises into your routine, maintain proper form, gradually increase resistance, and prioritize rest and recovery. By focusing on your core, lower back, hips, and legs, you're taking proactive steps to reduce sciatica pain, prevent future episodes, and regain control over your life.

In the chapters ahead, we'll explore cardiovascular exercises, low-impact options, and lifestyle modifications to complement your strengthening routine. With each strengthening exercise, you're building a more resilient and pain-free future. So, let's continue this journey with determination and optimism, knowing that you're

making significant strides toward
a more comfortable and active
lifestyle.

CHAPTER 7

Cardiovascular and Low-Impact Exercises

Welcome to Chapter 7, where we'll explore the role of cardiovascular and low-impact exercises in managing sciatica. Cardiovascular exercises get your heart pumping, while low-impact options offer the benefits of physical activity without placing excessive strain on your joints. These exercises are like the steady rhythm of your favorite song, helping reduce inflammation, improve circulation, and enhance overall well-being. In this chapter, we'll dive into the importance of these exercise categories, their benefits for sciatica, and specific activities to consider.

The Importance of Cardiovascular Exercise:

Cardiovascular exercises, often referred to as cardio or aerobic exercises, are activities that increase your heart rate and breathing. They play a pivotal role in maintaining overall health by promoting cardiovascular fitness, improving lung function, and aiding in weight management. But what does this have to do with managing sciatica?

Cardiovascular exercises have several indirect benefits for individuals with sciatica:

1. **Reduced Inflammation:** Cardio exercises help reduce inflammation in the body, which can alleviate sciatica symptoms, as inflammation often contributes to nerve irritation.

2. **Improved Circulation:** These exercises enhance blood flow, delivering essential nutrients and

oxygen to the affected area, which can aid in healing.

3. **Weight Management:** Maintaining a healthy weight is crucial for individuals with sciatica, as excess weight can exacerbate pain. Cardio helps with weight management.

4. **Mood Enhancement:** Cardio workouts trigger the release of endorphins, which can boost your mood and reduce stress – factors that can exacerbate sciatica pain.

Benefits of Cardiovascular Exercise for Sciatica:

Engaging in cardiovascular exercises offers numerous advantages for individuals dealing with sciatica:

1. **Pain Relief:** The reduced inflammation and improved circulation associated with cardio can help alleviate sciatica pain.

2. **Weight Management:** Cardio exercises assist in weight management, which can reduce the strain on the lower back and sciatic nerve.

3. **Enhanced Mobility:** Improved cardiovascular fitness can enhance your

overall mobility and reduce the risk of stiffness and discomfort.

4. **Mood Improvement:** Cardio workouts promote a sense of well-being and can help reduce the emotional impact of chronic pain.

The Low-Impact Alternative:

While cardiovascular exercises are beneficial, some individuals with sciatica may find high-impact activities, such as running or jumping, uncomfortable or painful. This is where low-impact exercises step in.

Low-impact exercises offer a gentler way to achieve cardiovascular benefits without putting excessive stress on the joints. These activities are like a gentle stream, flowing smoothly without causing turbulence. They can be particularly valuable for individuals with acute or chronic sciatica, joint issues, or those who are new to exercise.

Benefits of Low-Impact Exercise for Sciatica:

Low-impact exercises provide several advantages for sciatica management:

1. **Joint-Friendly:** These exercises are gentle on the joints, reducing the risk of aggravating pain or causing injury.

2. **Improved Circulation:** Like cardio exercises, low-impact activities enhance blood flow and circulation, aiding in healing and reducing inflammation.

3. **Enhanced Flexibility:** Many low-impact exercises, such as swimming and tai chi, incorporate gentle stretching, improving flexibility and reducing muscle tension.

4. **Reduced Stress:** The low-impact nature of these activities can help lower stress levels, which is beneficial for managing sciatica-related discomfort.

Cardiovascular and Low-Impact Exercises for Sciatica:

Now, let's explore specific cardiovascular and low-impact exercises that can benefit individuals with sciatica. As always, it's crucial to start gradually, listen to your body, and consult with a healthcare professional if you have any concerns about your exercise routine.

Cardiovascular Exercises:

1. **Walking:** A simple yet effective cardiovascular exercise, walking is a low-impact activity that you can tailor to your fitness level. Start with short walks and gradually increase the duration.

2. **Swimming:** Swimming and water aerobics are excellent choices for sciatica management. The buoyancy of water reduces impact on

joints while providing a full-body workout.

3. **Cycling:** Stationary or outdoor cycling is a great option for cardiovascular fitness. Ensure that your bike is properly fitted to minimize strain on your lower back.

4. **Elliptical Trainer:** The elliptical machine provides a low-impact, full-body workout. It's an excellent choice for individuals with sciatica as it minimizes joint stress.

Low-Impact Exercises:

1. **Tai Chi:** This ancient Chinese practice combines gentle, flowing movements with deep breathing. It improves balance, flexibility, and strength while being easy on the joints.

2. **Yoga:** Many yoga poses and sequences focus on stretching and strengthening the lower back, hips, and core. Choose gentle or beginner-level classes to start.

3. **Pilates:** Pilates emphasizes core strength, flexibility, and body awareness. It's especially effective for

strengthening the muscles that support the spine.

4. **Stationary Rowing:** Using a rowing machine provides a full-body, low-impact workout. It engages the legs, core, and upper body while minimizing stress on the lower back.

Pre-Exercise Guidelines:

Before engaging in any cardiovascular or low-impact exercise routine, it's important to consider these guidelines:

1. **Consult with a Healthcare Professional:**

If you have any doubts or underlying medical conditions, consult with a healthcare provider before starting a new exercise regimen.

2. **Proper Warm-Up:** Begin with a 5-10 minute warm-up to prepare your muscles and joints for exercise. Light cardio, such as brisk walking or cycling, is a good choice.

3. **Gradual Progression:** Start at a comfortable level and gradually increase the intensity and duration

CHAPTER 8

Lifestyle Modifications for Sciatica Relief

Welcome to Chapter 8, where we'll explore the significance of lifestyle modifications in managing sciatica. Your lifestyle is like the canvas on which you paint your well-being, and by making thoughtful changes, you can create an environment that promotes healing, reduces pain, and supports your overall health. In this chapter, we'll discuss how lifestyle factors, including posture, ergonomics, nutrition, and stress management, play a crucial role in your journey toward sciatica relief.

The Impact of Lifestyle on Sciatica:

Imagine your lifestyle as the stage where the drama of your health unfolds. The way you live, move, and nourish your body can either alleviate or exacerbate sciatica pain. Understanding this influence empowers you to make choices that contribute to your well-being.

1. Posture:

Poor posture is like a misaligned puzzle piece – it can create discomfort and hinder your body's natural alignment. For individuals with sciatica, improper posture can increase the strain on the lower back and exacerbate pain. Here's how to maintain better posture:

- When sitting, keep your feet flat on the floor, knees at hip level, and back supported. Consider using a lumbar cushion for additional support.
- While standing, distribute your weight evenly on both feet and engage your core

muscles to support your spine.

- When lifting objects, bend at the knees and hips, not the waist, to reduce strain on your lower back.

2. Ergonomics:

Your work environment can significantly impact your sciatica. Whether you work from an office or home, ensuring proper ergonomics is essential. Consider these tips:

- Use an ergonomic chair with lumbar support to maintain good posture while working.

- Adjust the height of your computer screen so that it's at eye level to reduce strain on your neck and upper back.
- Take regular breaks to stand, stretch, and walk around if you have a sedentary job.

3. Nutrition:

Nutrition is the fuel that powers your body's functions, including the healing process. Maintaining a balanced diet can help reduce inflammation, support tissue repair, and contribute to overall well-being:

- Incorporate anti-inflammatory foods like fruits, vegetables, fatty fish (rich in omega-3s), nuts, and seeds into your diet.
- Stay hydrated by drinking plenty of water, which helps in maintaining spinal discs' hydration.
- Limit or avoid foods high in sugar and processed fats, as they can promote inflammation.

4. Exercise and Movement:

Exercise, as we've discussed in previous chapters, is a crucial component of sciatica management. Regular physical activity keeps your muscles and joints healthy, improves circulation, and reduces inflammation.

- Incorporate both stretching and strengthening exercises into your routine to address muscle imbalances and support the spine.
- Engage in cardiovascular or low-impact exercises to improve overall fitness and reduce pain.

5. Stress Management:

Stress is like a storm that can worsen the waters of sciatica pain. Chronic stress can lead to muscle tension and inflammation, exacerbating sciatica symptoms. Strategies to manage stress include:

- Practicing relaxation techniques such as deep breathing, meditation, or yoga.
- Prioritizing self-care and engaging in activities you enjoy to reduce stress levels.
- Seeking support from a therapist or counselor if stress and pain are

significantly impacting your quality of life.

6. Sleep:

Sleep is the body's natural healer, and quality rest is vital for managing sciatica. Poor sleep can worsen pain perception and slow the healing process.

- Invest in a comfortable mattress and pillows that support your spine and promote a neutral sleeping posture.
- Maintain a regular sleep schedule, aiming for 7-9 hours of sleep per night.

7. Footwear:

Your choice of footwear can influence the way you walk and stand, affecting your posture and potentially contributing to sciatica pain.

- Wear supportive, comfortable shoes that provide arch support and cushioning.
- Avoid high heels or shoes with inadequate arch support for extended periods.

8. Smoking:

Smoking can hinder the body's ability to heal and reduce blood flow, potentially worsening sciatica symptoms.

- Consider quitting smoking to improve circulation and overall health.

9. Weight Management:

Excess weight can increase the load on your spine and exacerbate sciatica pain. Maintaining a healthy weight through diet and exercise is essential for long-term relief.

10. Avoid Prolonged Sitting:

Sitting for extended periods can put pressure on the lower back and sciatic nerve. If you have a desk job, make a point to stand, stretch, and walk briefly every hour.

11. Listen to Your Body:

Above all, it's essential to listen to your body. Pay attention to how specific activities or postures affect your pain. If something exacerbates your symptoms, consider modifying or avoiding it.

Consulting with Healthcare Professionals:

While lifestyle modifications are valuable, they should complement, not replace, medical advice and treatment. If you're struggling with severe or persistent sciatica pain, it's crucial to consult with healthcare professionals who can provide tailored guidance and interventions.

- A primary care physician can evaluate your condition and recommend appropriate treatments, including medications or referrals to specialists.
- A physical therapist can design a personalized

exercise program and provide techniques for pain relief.

- An orthopedic specialist or neurologist may be consulted for more complex cases or if surgical intervention is considered.

The Holistic Approach:

Managing sciatica is not a one-size-fits-all endeavor. It's a holistic journey that combines exercise, lifestyle modifications, and medical guidance to reduce pain and improve overall well-being. By addressing various aspects of your life, you can create an environment that fosters healing and empowers you to regain control over your health.

Closing Thoughts:

Chapter 8 has explored the role of lifestyle modifications in managing sciatica. Your lifestyle choices significantly influence your well-being and can either alleviate or exacerbate sciatica pain. By making thoughtful changes in areas such as posture, ergonomics, nutrition,

CONCLUSION

In conclusion, the journey through this book has been a comprehensive exploration of sciatica and its management through exercise and lifestyle adjustments. Sciatica, often caused by irritation of the sciatic nerve, can lead to debilitating pain and discomfort. However, armed with knowledge and a tailored approach, individuals can regain control over their well-being and find relief from sciatic pain.

Throughout the eight chapters of this book, we've covered a wide range of topics:

1. **Understanding Sciatica:** We began by comprehending the nature of sciatica, its causes, and its impact on daily life.

2. **Anatomy and Sciatica:** We explored the anatomy of the spine and the sciatic nerve, providing a foundation for understanding the root causes of sciatica.

3. **Types of Sciatica:** We delved into the different

types of sciatica and their specific triggers, enabling readers to identify their condition accurately.

4. **Preparing for Exercise:** We emphasized the importance of assessment, seeking professional guidance, setting realistic goals, and understanding pain signals before embarking on an exercise regimen.

5. **Stretching and Flexibility:** We learned how stretching and flexibility exercises can alleviate tension, reduce

muscle imbalances, and contribute to sciatica relief.

6. **Strengthening Exercises:** We explored strengthening exercises that target key muscle groups to provide support for the spine and minimize pressure on the sciatic nerve.

7. **Cardiovascular and Low-Impact Exercises:** We discovered how cardiovascular and low-impact exercises contribute to overall health, reduce inflammation, and enhance well-being for individuals with sciatica.

8. **Lifestyle Modifications:**
Finally, we explored the role of lifestyle adjustments, including posture, ergonomics, nutrition, stress management, sleep, and more, in managing and preventing sciatica.

By combining the insights from these chapters, individuals can develop a holistic approach to managing their sciatica. It begins with understanding their condition, seeking professional guidance, and adopting a tailored exercise routine that encompasses stretching, strengthening, cardiovascular activities, and low-impact exercises. Additionally, making mindful lifestyle modifications, such as maintaining proper posture, staying active, managing stress, and supporting overall health, contributes to a comprehensive strategy for pain relief.

It's important to note that everyone's journey is unique. Consultation with healthcare professionals, personalized exercise plans, and adaptation to individual needs and limitations are key factors in achieving optimal results. With dedication, consistency, and the knowledge acquired from this book, individuals can pave the way to a life with reduced sciatica pain, improved mobility, and enhanced well-being.

Remember, this book is not the end of your journey; it's a stepping stone toward better health. As you move forward, continue to learn, adapt, and prioritize your well-being. Sciatica management is about empowerment, and armed with the knowledge you've gained, you are well-equipped to take control of your health and lead a more comfortable and active life.

9 798864 060551